M.T. EDWARD

Mastering Medicare

An Essential Guide for Maximizing Your Coverage

Contents

Introduction

Welcome to "Mastering Medicare: An Essential Guide for Maximizing Your Coverage." If you're reading this, congratulations are in order – you're about to embark on a journey towards understanding one of the most crucial aspects of your healthcare coverage. Medicare can be a complex maze, but fear not, for this book is designed to be your trusty compass, guiding you through its intricacies with ease and clarity.

In this introductory chapter, we'll lay the groundwork for what lies ahead. We'll discuss why it's essential to grasp the ins and outs of Medicare, particularly for those new to the program. Whether you're approaching the age of 65 or qualifying due to social security disability, navigating Medicare can feel daunting. However, armed with the right knowledge, you'll soon discover that it's not as intimidating as it seems.

We'll start by providing a brief overview of the four main parts of Medicare: Parts A, B, C, and D. These components form the backbone of your coverage, each serving a unique purpose in safeguarding your health and financial well-being. But don't worry; we won't drown you in jargon or technicalities. Our aim is to simplify these concepts, making them accessible to readers of all backgrounds.

The purpose of this book is straightforward: to demystify Medicare and empower you to make informed decisions about your healthcare. Whether you're looking to understand your current coverage better or preparing to enroll for the first time, this guide has you covered. Each chapter is crafted with care, offering practical advice and actionable steps to help you maximize your benefits and navigate the system with confidence.

So, how should you approach this guide? Think of it as your go-to resource, a companion on your Medicare journey. Whether you read it cover to cover or jump straight to the sections that pique your interest, the choice is yours. Our goal is simple: to equip you with the knowledge and tools you need to master Medicare and take control of your healthcare destiny.

With that said, let's dive in and begin unraveling the mysteries of Medicare. Your path to mastering your coverage starts here.

1

Original Medicare

In this chapter, we'll delve into the cornerstone of Medicare: Original Medicare. We'll explore the ins and outs of Part A hospital coverage and Part B medical coverage, shedding light on what's included, what's not, and crucial timelines for enrollment.

Part A - Hospital Coverage

Welcome to the heart of your Medicare coverage: Part A hospital coverage. This essential component ensures you have access to necessary hospital services, including inpatient care, skilled nursing facility care, hospice care, and some home health care. We'll walk you through what each of these services entails, giving you a clear understanding of the safety net Original Medicare provides in times of medical need.

Part B - Medical Coverage

Next up, we'll explore Part B medical coverage, which plays a vital role in covering outpatient services, preventive care, durable medical equipment, and more. From doctor visits to lab tests, Part B has you covered when it comes to maintaining your health and well-being outside of a hospital setting. We'll break down the specifics of what's included and how to make the most of your Part B benefits.

What Original Medicare Doesn't Cover

While Original Medicare provides comprehensive coverage for many healthcare services, it's essential to understand its limitations. In this section, we'll outline what Original Medicare doesn't cover, from prescription drugs to dental and vision care. By knowing what gaps exist in your coverage, you can take proactive steps to fill them through other means, such as supplemental insurance or Medicare Advantage plans.

When to Enroll and What to Expect After Enrollment

Timing is everything when it comes to enrolling in Original Medicare. We'll guide you through the enrollment process, highlighting key deadlines and considerations based on your unique circumstances. Additionally, we'll discuss what to expect after enrolling in Original Medicare, including how to access your benefits, pay premiums, and navigate any initial hurdles that may arise.

Part A - Hospital Coverage

Welcome to the cornerstone of your Medicare coverage: Part A hospital coverage. Part A ensures you have access to essential hospital services, providing peace of mind in times of medical need. Here's a detailed overview of what Part A covers:

Inpatient Hospital Care:

- Part A covers your stay in a hospital as an inpatient, including a semi-private room, meals, general nursing, and other hospital services and supplies. This includes necessary medical procedures, surgeries, and treatments administered during your hospital stay.

Skilled Nursing Facility (SNF) Care:

- If you require skilled nursing care or rehabilitation services following a hospital stay, Part A may cover your stay in a skilled nursing facility. This includes services such as physical therapy, occupational therapy, and speech-language pathology services.

Hospice Care:

- Part A provides coverage for hospice care if you have a terminal illness and have chosen to receive palliative care to manage symptoms and improve quality of life. This includes medical and support services for both the patient and their family members.

Home Health Care:

- Part A covers medically necessary home health services, including skilled nursing care, physical therapy, occupational therapy, speech-language pathology services, and medical social services. This allows you to receive necessary medical care in the comfort of your own home.

Blood Transfusions:

- Part A covers the cost of blood transfusions received during a covered inpatient stay, up to a certain limit.

It's important to note that while Part A provides coverage for many hospital-related services, it may not cover all costs associated with your care. You may be responsible for deductibles, coinsurance, and other out-of-pocket expenses. Additionally, certain services may have limitations or eligibility criteria, so it's essential to familiarize yourself with the specifics of your Part A coverage.

Understanding Part A hospital coverage is the first step towards making informed decisions about your healthcare. By knowing what services are covered under Part A, you can confidently navigate the healthcare system and access the care you need when you need it most.

Part B - Medical Coverage

Welcome to Part B medical coverage, an essential component of your Medicare benefits. Part B ensures you have access to a wide range of medical services outside of a hospital setting, helping you stay healthy and proactive in managing your healthcare needs. Here's a detailed overview of what Part B covers:

Doctor Visits:

- Part B covers visits to doctors, specialists, and other healthcare providers for medically necessary services, including consultations, examinations, and treatments.

Outpatient Care:

- Part B provides coverage for outpatient services and procedures, such as diagnostic tests, X-rays, laboratory services, and medical equipment used outside of a hospital.

Preventive Services:

- Part B covers a variety of preventive services aimed at maintaining your health and detecting potential health issues early. This includes screenings for cancer, diabetes, cardiovascular disease, and other conditions, as well as vaccinations and counseling services.

Durable Medical Equipment (DME):

- Part B helps cover the cost of durable medical equipment, such as wheelchairs, walkers, hospital beds, and oxygen equipment, that is deemed medically necessary for your treatment or mobility.

Ambulance Services:

- Part B provides coverage for ambulance services when other transportation could endanger your health, and the transportation is necessary to obtain medical care.

Mental Health Services:

- Part B covers certain mental health services, including outpatient therapy and counseling sessions with licensed mental health professionals.

Second Opinion Before Surgery:

- Part B allows you to seek a second opinion from a different doctor before undergoing non-emergency surgery. Medicare will generally cover the cost of this second opinion.

Understanding what Part B covers is essential for making informed decisions about your healthcare. By taking advantage of the services covered under Part B, you can proactively manage your health and address any medical concerns that may arise. Keep in mind that while Part B provides comprehensive coverage for many medical services, you may be responsible for deductibles, coinsurance, and other out-of-pocket expenses. Be sure to review your Part B coverage carefully to understand your rights and responsibilities as a Medicare beneficiary.

What Original Medicare Doesn't Cover

While Original Medicare provides comprehensive coverage for many healthcare services, it's essential to be aware of its limitations. Here's a detailed overview of what Original Medicare doesn't cover:

Prescription Drugs:

- Original Medicare (Parts A and B) generally does not cover prescription drugs you take at home. However, you can obtain prescription drug coverage through Medicare Part D, a standalone prescription drug plan, or a Medicare Advantage plan that includes prescription drug coverage, which we will cover in the subsequent chapters.

Dental Care:

- Routine dental care, including cleanings, fillings, extractions, and dentures, is not covered by Original Medicare. You may need to consider separate dental insurance or discount plans to help cover these costs.

Vision Care:

- Original Medicare does not cover routine eye exams, eyeglasses, or contact lenses. However, it may cover certain medically necessary eye exams and treatments for eye diseases or conditions.

Hearing Aids and Exams:

- Original Medicare does not cover hearing exams or hearing aids. However, it may cover diagnostic hearing and balance exams if your doctor orders them to diagnose or treat a medical condition.

Long-Term Care:

- Original Medicare does not cover most long-term care services, including assistance with activities of daily living (such as bathing, dressing, and eating) in a nursing home or at home. You may need to explore long-term care insurance or Medicaid for coverage of these services.

Cosmetic Surgery:

- Original Medicare does not cover cosmetic procedures or surgeries performed solely for aesthetic reasons.

Acupuncture:

- Original Medicare typically does not cover acupuncture for most conditions. However, there are some limited exceptions for certain chronic pain conditions.

Routine Foot Care:

- Original Medicare does not cover routine foot care, such as nail trimming or callus removal, unless it is related to a medical condition such as diabetes.

Medical Care Received Outside the United States:

- Original Medicare generally does not cover medical care received outside the United States, except in limited situations such as emergencies.

Understanding what Original Medicare doesn't cover is crucial for planning your healthcare needs effectively. While Original Medicare provides essential coverage for many services, it's essential to explore additional coverage options, such as Medicare Advantage plans or supplemental insurance, to fill in the gaps and ensure comprehensive care. Be sure to review your Medicare coverage carefully and consider your individual healthcare needs when making decisions about additional coverage.

When to Enroll and How

Understanding when and how to enroll in Original Medicare is essential for ensuring seamless access to healthcare benefits. Here's a comprehensive guide to help you navigate the enrollment process:

Initial Enrollment Period (IEP):

- For most individuals, the Initial Enrollment Period (IEP) begins three months before the month of your 65th birthday and ends three months after the month you turn 65. During this seven-month period, you have the opportunity to enroll in Original Medicare (Parts A and B) without incurring any late enrollment penalties.

Special Enrollment Periods (SEPs):

- Certain circumstances may qualify you for a Special Enrollment Period (SEP) outside of the IEP. These include situations such as continuing to work past age 65 with employer-sponsored health coverage, moving outside of your plan's service area, or qualifying for Medicare due to a disability.

General Enrollment Period (GEP):

- If you miss your Initial Enrollment Period, you can enroll in Original Medicare during the General Enrollment Period (GEP), which runs from January 1st to March 31st each year. However, late enrollment penalties may apply, and coverage may not begin until July 1st of that year.

How to Enroll:

- Enrolling in Original Medicare is typically an automatic process if you're already receiving Social Security benefits. In this case, you'll be enrolled in Parts A and B automatically and will receive your Medicare card in the mail about three months before your 65th birthday.
- If you're not yet receiving Social Security benefits, you'll need to actively enroll in Medicare. You can do this online through the Social Security Administration's website, by visiting your local Social Security office, or by calling Social Security's toll-free number.

Consider Additional Coverage:

- While Original Medicare provides essential coverage, it may not cover all of your healthcare needs. Consider enrolling in Medicare

Part D for prescription drug coverage and explore options for supplemental coverage such as Medicare Supplement Insurance (Medigap) or Medicare Advantage plans to help fill in the gaps. We will cover these products in the following chapters.

By understanding when to enroll and how to navigate the enrollment process, you can ensure timely access to the healthcare benefits provided by Original Medicare. Be sure to familiarize yourself with enrollment deadlines and explore additional coverage options to tailor your healthcare coverage to your individual needs effectively.

What to Expect After Enrollment

Congratulations on enrolling in Original Medicare! Now that you've taken this important step towards securing your healthcare coverage, it's essential to understand what to expect next. Here's a guide to help you navigate life after enrollment:

Medicare Card Arrival:

- After enrolling in Original Medicare, you can expect to receive your Medicare card in the mail within three weeks. This card will include your Medicare number and the dates your coverage begins.

Premiums and Deductibles:

- Depending on your work history, you may not have to pay a premium for Medicare Part A (hospital insurance). However, most people pay a monthly premium for Medicare Part B (medical insurance). You'll receive a bill for your Part B premium every month.
- Original Medicare also has deductibles and coinsurance amounts that you may be responsible for paying out of pocket. Familiarize

yourself with these costs to budget accordingly for your healthcare expenses.

Coverage Start Date:

- Your Medicare coverage will typically begin on the first day of the month you turn 65 if you enrolled during your Initial Enrollment Period. If you enrolled later, your coverage start date may vary.

Using Your Benefits:

- Once your Medicare coverage begins, you can start using your benefits right away. Schedule any necessary doctor's appointments, screenings, or medical procedures knowing that your Medicare coverage will help cover the costs.

Understanding Coverage:

- Take the time to review your Medicare coverage documents carefully. Understand what services are covered, what costs you may be responsible for, and any limitations or exclusions that may apply.

Prescription Drug Coverage:

- If you enrolled in a Medicare Part D prescription drug plan or a Medicare Advantage plan with prescription drug coverage, you'll receive a separate card for your prescription drug benefits. Use this card when filling prescriptions at the pharmacy.

Explore Additional Coverage Options:

- Consider exploring additional coverage options to enhance your Medicare benefits. This may include enrolling in a Medicare Supplement Insurance (Medigap) plan to help cover out-of-pocket costs or joining a Medicare Advantage plan for comprehensive coverage.

By knowing what to expect after enrolling in Original Medicare, you can transition smoothly into using your benefits and accessing the healthcare services you need. Stay informed, keep your Medicare card handy, and don't hesitate to reach out to Medicare or your healthcare provider if you have any questions or concerns along the way.

2

Part C - Medicare Advantage

Welcome to the world of Medicare Advantage plans. This chapter is designed to provide you with a comprehensive understanding of Medicare Advantage, including how it works alongside Original Medicare, the different types of plans available, and tips for selecting the right plan for your needs.

Overview of Medicare Advantage Plans

In this section, we'll provide an in-depth overview of Medicare Advantage plans, also known as Medicare Part C. We'll explore how these plans differ from Original Medicare, the various types of coverage they offer, and the benefits of choosing a Medicare Advantage plan.

How it Coordinates with Medicare Part A and Part B

Understanding how Medicare Advantage plans coordinate with Medicare Parts A and B is crucial for maximizing your coverage. We'll delve into the relationship between Medicare Advantage and Original Medicare, including how benefits are provided and potential cost-saving opportunities.

Health Maintenance Organization (HMO) Plans

Health Maintenance Organization (HMO) plans are one type of Medicare Advantage plan. We'll take a closer look at how HMO plans operate, including their network restrictions, primary care physician requirements, and potential advantages and disadvantages.

Preferred Provider Organization (PPO) Plans

Preferred Provider Organization (PPO) plans offer another option for Medicare beneficiaries. We'll explore the flexibility and freedom of choice that PPO plans provide, as well as their cost-sharing structure and considerations for selecting a PPO plan.

Why You Should Enroll in a Medicare Advantage Plan

In this section, we'll highlight the benefits of enrolling in a Medicare Advantage plan, including enhanced coverage options, additional benefits such as prescription drug coverage and dental care, and potential cost savings compared to Original Medicare.

Pros and Cons of Medicare Advantage Plans

We'll provide a balanced overview of the pros and cons of Medicare Advantage plans, helping you weigh the advantages of additional benefits and cost savings against potential limitations such as network restrictions and out-of-pocket costs.

How to Shop for the Right Plan

Selecting the right Medicare Advantage plan requires careful consideration of your healthcare needs and preferences. We'll offer practical tips and strategies for comparing plans, evaluating coverage options, and choosing the plan that best fits your individual circumstances.

When You Can Enroll and How

Understanding the enrollment process for Medicare Advantage plans is essential for securing coverage when you need it. We'll outline the various enrollment periods, including Initial Enrollment, Annual Enrollment, and Special Enrollment periods, and explain how to enroll in a Medicare Advantage plan.

Overview of Medicare Advantage Plans

Let's start with an overview of Medicare Advantage plans, an alternative way to receive your Medicare benefits. Medicare Advantage plans, also known as Medicare Part C, are offered by private insurance companies approved by Medicare. These plans provide all of your Part A (hospital insurance) and Part B (medical insurance) coverage and often include additional benefits such as prescription drug coverage, vision, dental, and hearing care. Medicare Advantage plans may also offer coverage for services not covered by Original Medicare, like gym memberships or telehealth services. With Medicare Advantage, you receive your benefits through the plan, and most plans require you to use a network of doctors and hospitals. These plans typically have a monthly premium, in addition to any premiums you pay for Medicare Part B. By enrolling in a Medicare Advantage plan, you can enjoy comprehensive coverage and potentially save on out-of-pocket costs compared to Original Medicare.

How it Coordinates with Medicare Part A and Part B

Understanding how Medicare Advantage plans coordinate with Medicare Parts A and B is essential for maximizing your coverage. Medicare Advantage plans essentially take the place of Original Medicare (Parts A and B) and provide all of the same benefits, plus potentially additional benefits. When you enroll in a Medicare Advantage plan, you're still part of the Medicare program, but you receive your benefits through the private insurance company that administers your plan.

Here's how it works:

Medicare Part A Coverage:

- Your Medicare Advantage plan will cover all of the hospital services that Medicare Part A covers. This includes inpatient hospital care, skilled nursing facility care, hospice care, and some home health care services. However, the specific rules and coverage details may vary depending on the plan you choose.

Medicare Part B Coverage:

- Similarly, your Medicare Advantage plan will cover all of the medical services that Medicare Part B covers. This includes doctor's visits, outpatient care, preventive services, durable medical equipment, and more. Again, the coverage specifics may vary by plan.

Additional Benefits:

- In addition to the benefits provided by Original Medicare, many Medicare Advantage plans offer additional benefits such as prescription drug coverage, vision, dental, and hearing care. Some plans may also include coverage for services not covered by Original Medicare, like fitness programs or telehealth services.

It's important to note that while Medicare Advantage plans must provide at least the same level of coverage as Original Medicare, they may have different rules, costs, and restrictions. For example, most Medicare Advantage plans require you to use a network of doctors and hospitals, and you may need a referral from your primary care physician to see a specialist.

By understanding how Medicare Advantage plans coordinate with Medicare Parts A and B, you can make an informed decision about whether a Medicare Advantage plan is right for you and choose a plan that meets your healthcare needs and preferences.

Why You Should Enroll in a Medicare Advantage Plan

Enrolling in a Medicare Advantage plan offers several potential benefits that may make it a wise choice for many Medicare beneficiaries. Here's why you should consider enrolling in a Medicare Advantage plan:

Comprehensive Coverage:

- Medicare Advantage plans often provide all of the benefits covered by Original Medicare (Parts A and B) and may include additional benefits such as prescription drug coverage, vision, dental, and hearing care. By enrolling in a Medicare Advantage plan, you can access a wide range of healthcare services under one comprehensive plan.

Additional Benefits:

- Many Medicare Advantage plans offer extra benefits that aren't covered by Original Medicare, such as fitness programs, transportation services, and telehealth visits. These added benefits can enhance your overall healthcare experience and help you maintain your health and well-being.

Cost Savings:

- Medicare Advantage plans may offer cost-saving opportunities compared to Original Medicare. While you'll still pay your Medicare Part B premium, Medicare Advantage plans often have lower monthly premiums and out-of-pocket costs, such as copayments and coinsurance. Additionally, some plans may offer coverage for services like prescription drugs with lower or no additional cost-sharing.

Coordination of Care:

- Medicare Advantage plans often provide coordinated care through a network of healthcare providers. This means that your primary care physician (PCP) can help manage your healthcare needs and coordinate referrals to specialists, ensuring that you receive comprehensive and well-coordinated care.

Flexibility:

- Depending on the type of Medicare Advantage plan you choose, you may have flexibility in choosing your healthcare providers and accessing care outside of the plan's network. This flexibility can be particularly beneficial if you travel frequently or have specific healthcare providers you prefer to see.

Convenience:

- Medicare Advantage plans typically offer one-stop shopping for all of your healthcare needs. With a single plan, you can access coverage for hospital stays, doctor visits, prescription drugs, and more, simplifying the process of managing your healthcare benefits.

Overall, enrolling in a Medicare Advantage plan can offer comprehensive coverage, additional benefits, potential cost savings, coordinated care, flexibility, and convenience. By carefully evaluating your healthcare needs and comparing available plans, you can make an informed decision about whether a Medicare Advantage plan is the right choice for you.

Health Maintenance Organization (HMO) Plans

Health Maintenance Organization (HMO) plans are a type of Medicare Advantage plan that offers comprehensive coverage within a network of healthcare providers. Here's a detailed yet simplified description of how HMO plans work:

Network of Providers:

- HMO plans have a network of doctors, hospitals, and other healthcare providers that you must use for your care. These providers have agreed to offer services to plan members at a predetermined cost.

Primary Care Physician (PCP):

- With an HMO plan, you'll typically choose a primary care physician (PCP) from within the plan's network. Your PCP will be your main point of contact for all of your healthcare needs and will coordinate your care, including referrals to specialists if needed.

Referrals:

- In most cases, you'll need a referral from your PCP to see a specialist or receive certain medical services. This helps ensure that your care is coordinated and that you're receiving the appropriate level of care for your needs.

Coverage for Out-of-Network Care:

- HMO plans generally do not cover care received outside of the plan's network, except in emergencies or other rare circumstances. If you choose to see an out-of-network provider without a referral, you may be responsible for the full cost of the services.

Cost Savings:

- HMO plans often have lower premiums and out-of-pocket costs compared to other types of Medicare Advantage plans. By staying within the plan's network and following the rules, you can potentially save money on your healthcare expenses.

Comprehensive Coverage:

- HMO plans typically offer comprehensive coverage for all of the benefits provided by Original Medicare (Parts A and B), as well as additional benefits such as prescription drug coverage and preventive services.

Overall, HMO plans offer a balance of affordability and comprehensive coverage within a structured network of providers. By understanding how HMO plans operate and following the rules of the plan, you can access high-quality healthcare while potentially saving money on your healthcare costs.

Preferred Provider Organization (PPO) Plans

Preferred Provider Organization (PPO) plans are another type of Medicare Advantage plan that offers flexibility and choice in healthcare providers. Here's a detailed yet simplified description of how PPO plans work:

Network of Providers:

- PPO plans have a network of doctors, hospitals, and other health-care providers, similar to HMO plans. However, unlike HMO plans, PPO plans allow you to see providers both inside and outside of the plan's network.

In-Network vs. Out-of-Network Coverage:

- With a PPO plan, you have the flexibility to see any healthcare provider you choose, whether they are in-network or out-of-network. However, you'll typically pay less for services received from providers within the plan's network.

No Referrals Required:

- Unlike HMO plans, PPO plans generally do not require referrals from a primary care physician (PCP) to see a specialist or receive certain medical services. You have the freedom to schedule appointments with specialists directly, without needing permission from your PCP.

Cost-sharing:

- While PPO plans offer more flexibility in choosing providers, they may have higher premiums and out-of-pocket costs compared to HMO plans. You'll typically pay a copayment or coinsurance for covered services, both in-network and out-of-network.

Coverage for Out-of-Network Care:

- PPO plans provide coverage for care received outside of the plan's network, although you may pay more for out-of-network services compared to in-network services. This flexibility can be valuable if you live in an area with limited network options or if you have specific healthcare providers you prefer to see.

Comprehensive Coverage:

- Like HMO plans, PPO plans offer comprehensive coverage for all of the benefits provided by Original Medicare (Parts A and B), as well as additional benefits such as prescription drug coverage and preventive services.

Overall, PPO plans offer the flexibility to see any healthcare provider you choose, both within and outside of the plan's network. By understanding how PPO plans operate and weighing the trade-offs between cost and flexibility, you can select a plan that meets your healthcare needs and preferences.

Pros and Cons of Medicare Advantage Plans

Medicare Advantage plans offer several advantages that make them an appealing option for many Medicare beneficiaries. One of the main benefits is the comprehensive coverage they provide, often including all of the benefits covered by Original Medicare (Parts A and B) along with additional benefits like prescription drug coverage, vision, dental, and hearing care. These added benefits can help individuals manage their health more effectively and may result in cost savings compared to Original Medicare. Another advantage of Medicare Advantage plans is the convenience they offer, with most plans providing one-stop shopping for all of your healthcare needs. Additionally, many Medicare Advantage plans provide coordinated care through a network of healthcare providers, ensuring that your healthcare needs are well-managed and that you receive timely and appropriate care.

However, Medicare Advantage plans also have some potential drawbacks that individuals should consider when making their decision. One downside is the limitations on provider choice, as most plans require you to use a network of doctors and hospitals. This restriction can be problematic if you have specific healthcare providers you prefer to see or if you live in an area with limited network options. Additionally, Medicare Advantage plans may have higher out-of-pocket costs for certain services, such as copayments and coinsurance, compared to Original Medicare. Finally, individuals enrolled in Medicare Advantage plans may face restrictions on coverage when seeking care outside of the plan's network, which can be a concern for those who travel frequently or have complex healthcare needs requiring specialized care. Overall, while Medicare Advantage plans offer comprehensive coverage and additional benefits, it's essential to weigh the pros and cons carefully to determine if a Medicare Advantage plan is the right choice for your individual healthcare needs and preferences.

How to Shop for the Right Plan

Shopping for the right Medicare Advantage plan can seem overwhelming, but by following some key steps and considerations, you can make an informed decision that meets your healthcare needs and preferences. Here are some best practices for shopping for a Medicare Advantage plan:

Assess Your Healthcare Needs:

- Start by evaluating your current healthcare needs, including any prescription medications you take, doctors you see regularly, and specific healthcare services you require. This will help you determine what benefits and coverage options are most important to you.

Compare Plan Options:

- Research and compare the Medicare Advantage plans available in your area. Look at factors such as premiums, deductibles, copayments, coinsurance, and out-of-pocket maximums. Pay attention to the plan's network of providers, prescription drug coverage, and additional benefits like vision, dental, and hearing care.

Consider Plan Types:

- Medicare Advantage plans come in different types, such as Health Maintenance Organization (HMO) plans, Preferred Provider Organization (PPO) plans, and Special Needs Plans (SNPs). Consider the pros and cons of each plan type and how they align with your healthcare preferences and provider preferences.

Review Plan Networks:

- Determine whether your current healthcare providers, including doctors, specialists, and hospitals, are included in the plan's network. If you have specific providers you prefer to see, make sure they participate in the plan to avoid unexpected out-of-network costs.

Evaluate Prescription Drug Coverage:

- If you take prescription medications, carefully review each plan's formulary to ensure that your medications are covered and that any restrictions or requirements (such as prior authorization or step therapy) align with your needs. Consider whether you need standalone prescription drug coverage (Medicare Part D) or if you prefer a Medicare Advantage plan with integrated drug coverage.

Consider Additional Benefits:

- Take note of any additional benefits offered by each plan, such as fitness programs, telehealth services, or vision and dental care. Determine whether these extra benefits are valuable to you and if they justify any additional costs associated with the plan.

Review Plan Ratings and Reviews:

- Check the quality ratings and customer reviews for each Medicare Advantage plan. Medicare assigns star ratings to plans based on factors such as quality of care, customer service, and member satisfaction. Additionally, read reviews from current plan members to get a sense of their experiences and satisfaction with the plan.

Seek Help if Needed:

- If you need assistance comparing plan options or understanding your coverage choices, consider reaching out to a licensed insurance agent, Medicare counselor, or the State Health Insurance Assistance Program (SHIP) for personalized assistance and guidance.

By following these best practices and taking the time to research and compare your options, you can find the Medicare Advantage plan that best fits your healthcare needs, preferences, and budget. Remember to review your plan annually during the Medicare Annual Enrollment Period (October 15 to December 7) to ensure that it continues to meet your needs as they evolve.

When You Can Enroll and How

Understanding when and how to enroll in a Medicare Advantage plan is essential for ensuring timely access to healthcare benefits. You have several opportunities to enroll in or make changes to your Medicare Advantage coverage:

Initial Enrollment Period (IEP):

- Your Initial Enrollment Period (IEP) for Medicare Advantage begins three months before the month you turn 65 and ends three months after your birthday month. During this seven-month period, you can enroll in a Medicare Advantage plan for the first time.

Annual Enrollment Period (AEP):

- The Annual Enrollment Period (AEP), also known as the Medicare Open Enrollment Period, occurs every year from October 15th to December 7th. During this time, you can switch or enroll in a Medicare Advantage plan, change your prescription drug coverage, or return to Original Medicare if you're enrolled in a Medicare Advantage plan.

Special Enrollment Periods (SEPs):

- Special Enrollment Periods (SEPs) may be available to individuals who experience qualifying life events, such as moving to a new area with different plan options, losing other healthcare coverage, or becoming eligible for Medicaid. SEPs allow you to enroll in or make changes to your Medicare Advantage coverage outside of the Initial Enrollment Period and Annual Enrollment Period.

To enroll in a Medicare Advantage plan, you can use several methods:

Online:

- Visit the Medicare website or the website of a private insurance company offering Medicare Advantage plans to explore plan options and enroll online.

By Phone:

- Call Medicare at 1-800-MEDICARE (1-800-633-4227) to speak with a representative who can help you enroll over the phone.

Through a Licensed Insurance Agent:

- Work with a licensed insurance agent who specializes in Medicare to discuss your options, compare plan features, and enroll in a Medicare Advantage plan that meets your needs.

In-Person:

- Visit a local insurance agent's office or attend a Medicare enrollment event in your community to receive assistance with enrolling in a Medicare Advantage plan.

When enrolling in a Medicare Advantage plan, be sure to have your Medicare card and any other relevant information, such as your preferred doctors and prescription medications, on hand. Take the time to carefully review plan details, including premiums, deductibles, copayments, and covered benefits, to select the plan that best fits your healthcare needs and budget. By understanding your enrollment options and taking advantage of available resources, you can enroll in a Medicare Advantage plan with confidence and ensure access to the healthcare coverage you need.

3

Medigap

Welcome to the world of Medicare supplement plans, also known as Medigap. This chapter is designed to provide you with a comprehensive understanding of how Medigap works alongside Original Medicare. We'll explore the different plan types, the pros, and cons of Medigap coverage, how to shop for the right plan, and the best time to enroll.

Overview of Medigap

In this section, we'll introduce Medigap and explain how it works with Original Medicare. We'll cover the basics of what Medigap plans are, how they supplement your Original Medicare coverage, and the benefits they provide.

Plan Types

We'll delve into the different types of Medigap plans available, including the standardized plan options offered in most states. We'll explain the coverage differences between each plan type and help you understand which plan may best meet your healthcare needs.

Pros and Cons of Medigap

This section will offer a balanced overview of the advantages and disadvantages of Medigap coverage. We'll explore the benefits of Medigap plans, such as comprehensive coverage and predictable out-of-pocket costs, as well as potential drawbacks like higher premiums and limited prescription drug coverage.

How to Know Which Plan is Right for You

We'll provide practical guidance on how to evaluate your healthcare needs and preferences to determine which Medigap plan is the best fit for you. We'll discuss factors to consider, such as your budget, healthcare usage patterns, and desired level of coverage.

Best Time to Enroll and How

Finally, we'll explain the best time to enroll in a Medigap plan and walk you through the enrollment process. We'll discuss key enrollment periods, such as the Initial Enrollment Period and Guaranteed Issue Rights and provide tips for navigating the enrollment process effectively.

Overview of Medigap

Medigap plans are designed to fill the "gaps" in coverage left by Original Medicare, providing additional financial protection and peace of mind for beneficiaries. These plans are offered by private insurance companies and are standardized across most states, meaning that the benefits provided by each plan type are consistent regardless of the insurance company offering the plan.

Medigap plans work alongside Original Medicare (Parts A and B) to help cover certain out-of-pocket costs, such as deductibles, copayments, and coinsurance. They do not typically cover services that Original Medicare does not cover, such as long-term care, vision, dental, hearing aids, or private-duty nursing. However, Medigap plans can provide financial assistance for Medicare-approved services, helping to reduce or eliminate your share of the costs.

There are several standardized Medigap plan types, labeled with letters from A to N, each offering a different level of coverage. Plan benefits are standardized by the federal government, so a Plan F from one insurance company will offer the same benefits as a Plan F from another company. However, premiums may vary depending on the insurance company, your location, and other factors.

When considering a Medigap plan, it's essential to assess your healthcare needs and budget carefully. Medigap plans can offer comprehensive coverage and predictable out-of-pocket costs, making them a popular choice for individuals who want financial protection and flexibility in choosing healthcare providers. However, Medigap plans may also have higher premiums compared to other coverage options, and they do not typically include prescription drug coverage.

Overall, Medigap plans can provide valuable supplemental coverage for Original Medicare beneficiaries, offering peace of mind and financial protection against unexpected healthcare costs. By understanding how Medigap works and comparing plan options, you can select a plan that meets your individual healthcare needs and budget.

Plan Types

Medigap plans are standardized across most states and are labeled with letters from A to N, each offering a different level of coverage. Here's a brief description of each plan type:

Plan A:

- Plan A provides basic coverage for essential benefits, including Medicare Part A coinsurance and hospital costs up to an additional

365 days after Medicare benefits are exhausted, Medicare Part B coinsurance or copayment, and the first three pints of blood each year.

Plan B:

- Similar to Plan A, Plan B offers basic coverage for essential benefits, including Medicare Part A coinsurance and hospital costs, Medicare Part B coinsurance or copayment, and the first three pints of blood each year. However, it also covers the Medicare Part A deductible.

Plan C:

- Plan C provides more comprehensive coverage, including all the benefits covered by Plan B, as well as coverage for Medicare Part B deductible and skilled nursing facility coinsurance.

Plan D:

- Plan D offers coverage for all the benefits covered by Plan C, except for the Medicare Part B deductible. It may be a suitable option for individuals looking for comprehensive coverage without coverage for the Part B deductible.

Plan F:

- Plan F is the most comprehensive Medigap plan, covering all the benefits covered by Plan C, as well as the Medicare Part B deductible. It offers the highest level of coverage and may be a good choice for individuals seeking minimal out-of-pocket costs.

Plan G:

- Plan G offers coverage similar to Plan F, except for the Medicare Part B deductible. It provides comprehensive coverage for all other benefits and may be a cost-effective alternative for individuals willing to pay the Part B deductible themselves.

Plan K:

- Plan K provides coverage for 50% of Medicare Part A coinsurance and hospital costs, as well as coverage for 50% of Medicare Part B coinsurance or copayment, hospice care coinsurance or copayment, and the first three pints of blood each year. It also has an out-of-pocket limit, after which the plan pays 100% of covered services for the rest of the year.

Plan L:

- Plan L offers coverage for 75% of Medicare Part A coinsurance and hospital costs, as well as coverage for 75% of Medicare Part B coinsurance or copayment, hospice care coinsurance or copayment, and the first three pints of blood each year. Like Plan K, it also has an out-of-pocket limit.

Plan M:

- Plan M provides coverage similar to Plan D, with the addition of coverage for 50% of the Medicare Part A deductible. It offers moderate coverage for essential benefits at a lower premium than more comprehensive plans.

Plan N:

- Plan N offers coverage similar to Plan D, with the addition of coverage for Medicare Part B coinsurance or copayment (excluding a copayment of up to $20 for some office visits and up to $50 for emergency room visits that don't result in inpatient admission). It provides comprehensive coverage with some cost-sharing for certain services.

Each plan type offers a different combination of coverage options and costs, allowing beneficiaries to choose the plan that best meets their healthcare needs and budget. It's essential to compare plan options carefully and consider factors such as premiums, coverage benefits, and out-of-pocket costs when selecting a Medigap plan.

Pros and Cons of Medigap

Medigap plans offer several advantages and disadvantages that individuals should consider when deciding whether to enroll in one. Here's an overview of the pros and cons of having a Medicare supplement plan:

Pros:

- Comprehensive Coverage: Medigap plans provide additional coverage beyond what Original Medicare offers, helping to fill in the "gaps" in coverage and providing financial protection against unexpected healthcare costs. With a Medigap plan, you can have peace of mind knowing that many of your out-of-pocket expenses, such as deductibles, copayments, and coinsurance, are covered.
- Predictable Costs: Medigap plans offer predictable out-of-pocket costs, making it easier to budget for healthcare expenses. Unlike

Original Medicare, which has coinsurance and copayments that can vary depending on the services you receive, Medigap plans typically have fixed costs that remain consistent throughout the year.

- Freedom to Choose Providers: With a Medigap plan, you have the freedom to choose any doctor, specialist, or hospital that accepts Medicare, without being restricted to a network of providers. This flexibility can be especially valuable if you have specific healthcare providers you prefer to see or if you travel frequently and need access to healthcare services outside of your local area.

- Coverage for Travel: Some Medigap plans offer coverage for emergency medical care when traveling outside of the United States, providing peace of mind for individuals who frequently travel internationally.

Cons:

- Higher Premiums: Medigap plans typically have higher monthly premiums compared to other types of Medicare coverage, such as Medicare Advantage plans. While the premiums may provide comprehensive coverage and predictable costs, they can be a financial burden for individuals on a fixed income or with limited resources.

- No Prescription Drug Coverage: Medigap plans do not typically include coverage for prescription drugs. Beneficiaries must enroll in a standalone Medicare Part D prescription drug plan to receive coverage for medications. This additional cost can increase overall healthcare expenses for individuals with high prescription drug costs.

- Limited Availability: Medigap plans are not available to everyone. To enroll in a Medigap plan, you must be enrolled in both Medicare Part A and Part B and live in the plan's service area. Additionally, insurance companies may use medical underwriting to determine eligibility or charge higher premiums based on your health status.

- Lack of Coverage for Additional Services: Medigap plans do not cover services that are not covered by Original Medicare, such as vision, dental, hearing aids, and long-term care. Beneficiaries may need to purchase separate insurance policies or pay out-of-pocket for these services.

Overall, Medigap plans offer comprehensive coverage and financial protection for Medicare beneficiaries, but they also come with higher premiums and limited coverage for certain services. It's essential to carefully consider your healthcare needs and budget when deciding whether a Medigap plan is the right choice for you.

Best Time to Enroll and How

Understanding the best time to enroll in a Medicare supplement plan, also known as Medigap, is crucial for ensuring access to coverage without facing penalties or restrictions. Here's an overview of the opportunities to enroll in a Medigap plan and how to do so:

Initial Enrollment Period (IEP):

- Your Initial Enrollment Period (IEP) for Medigap begins when you're both 65 years old and enrolled in Medicare Part B. This seven-month period provides the first opportunity to enroll in a Medigap plan without medical underwriting. During your IEP, insurance companies cannot deny you coverage or charge you higher premiums based on your health status.

Open Enrollment Period (OEP):

- If you miss your Initial Enrollment Period or choose to delay enrollment in a Medigap plan, you may have a second opportunity to enroll during the Open Enrollment Period (OEP). The OEP is a six-month period that begins when you're both 65 years old and enrolled in Medicare Part B. During this time, you have guaranteed-issue rights, meaning insurance companies cannot deny you coverage or charge you higher premiums due to pre-existing conditions.

Guaranteed-Issue Rights:

- In some situations, you may have guaranteed-issue rights to enroll in a Medigap plan without medical underwriting. For example, if you're losing employer-sponsored health coverage or your current Medigap plan is ending its coverage, you have a guaranteed right to purchase a new Medigap plan.

To enroll in a Medigap plan, you can follow these steps:

Research Plan Options:

- Research the available Medigap plans in your area and compare their coverage benefits, premiums, and customer ratings. You can use online resources, such as the Medicare website or insurance company websites, to explore plan options.

Contact Insurance Companies:

- Reach out to insurance companies offering Medigap plans in your area to request information and quotes. You can contact insurance companies directly by phone or visit their websites to request information online.

Compare Plan Costs and Benefits:

- Compare the costs and benefits of different Medigap plans to determine which plan best meets your healthcare needs and budget. Consider factors such as premiums, coverage benefits, and out-of-pocket costs when making your decision.

Enroll in a Plan:

- Once you've chosen a Medigap plan, you can enroll by completing an application with the insurance company offering the plan. You may need to provide information about your Medicare enrollment and personal details, such as your address and contact information.

Understand Waiting Periods:

- Keep in mind that some Medigap plans may have waiting periods for coverage of pre-existing conditions. Make sure you understand any waiting period requirements before enrolling in a plan.

By understanding the opportunities to enroll in a Medigap plan and following these steps, you can ensure access to comprehensive coverage and financial protection for your healthcare needs. If you have questions or need assistance with enrollment, consider reaching out to a licensed insurance agent or Medicare counselor for personalized guidance.

Frequently Asked Questions

Medicare members often have questions about Medicare supplement plans, or Medigap, as they navigate their healthcare coverage options. Here are some frequently asked questions (FAQs) from Medicare members about Medigap:

Can I switch Medigap plans or insurance companies?

- Yes, you have the flexibility to switch Medigap plans or insurance companies at any time. However, if you're outside of your Initial Enrollment Period or Open Enrollment Period, you may need to undergo medical underwriting, and insurance companies can deny you coverage or charge you higher premiums based on your health status.

Do Medigap plans cover prescription drugs?

- No, Medigap plans do not typically include coverage for prescription drugs. Beneficiaries must enroll in a standalone Medicare Part D prescription drug plan to receive coverage for medications. It's essential to consider your prescription drug needs when selecting a Medigap plan and Part D prescription drug plan.

Are Medigap premiums tax-deductible?

- In some cases, Medigap premiums may be tax-deductible if they exceed a certain percentage of your adjusted gross income (AGI). You should consult with a tax advisor or accountant to determine if you qualify for the deduction.

Can I have a Medicare Advantage plan and a Medigap plan at the same time?

- No, you cannot have both a Medicare Advantage plan and a Medigap plan at the same time. Medigap plans are designed to work alongside Original Medicare, while Medicare Advantage plans provide an alternative way to receive Medicare benefits. You must choose one type of coverage or the other.

Will my Medigap plan cover healthcare services received outside of the United States?

- Some Medigap plans offer coverage for emergency medical care when traveling outside of the United States. However, coverage is typically limited, and beneficiaries should carefully review their plan benefits and limitations before traveling internationally.

These are just a few of the frequently asked questions about Medicare supplement plans. If you have additional questions or need personalized assistance, consider reaching out to a licensed insurance agent, Medicare counselor, or the State Health Insurance Assistance Program (SHIP) for guidance.

4

Part D - Drug Coverage

Welcome to Part D of Medicare, where we delve into the world of prescription drug coverage. This chapter provides an essential overview of how Part D works, highlights the significance of having this coverage, and guides you through the enrollment process, including penalties and considerations.

Overview of Part D

In this section, we explore the fundamentals of Medicare Part D prescription drug coverage. We explain how Part D plans are offered by private insurance companies approved by Medicare, and how they help beneficiaries afford prescription medications. We also discuss the coverage gap (the "donut hole") and catastrophic coverage, key components of Part D plans.

Importance of Having Part D Coverage

Here, we emphasize the critical importance of having Medicare Part D coverage. We highlight how prescription medications play a vital role in managing health conditions and preventing costly complications.

We also discuss the financial protection that Part D provides, helping beneficiaries afford necessary medications and avoid high out-of-pocket costs.

How to Enroll

This section provides a step-by-step guide to enrolling in a Medicare Part D plan. We explain the different enrollment periods, including the Initial Enrollment Period (IEP), the Annual Enrollment Period (AEP), and Special Enrollment Periods (SEPs). We also discuss the various ways to enroll, such as through the Medicare website, over the phone, or with the assistance of a licensed insurance agent.

Late Enrollment Penalty

Here, we address the potential consequences of late enrollment in a Medicare Part D plan. We explain how beneficiaries may incur a late enrollment penalty if they go without creditable prescription drug coverage for a continuous period of 63 days or more after their Initial Enrollment Period ends. We provide guidance on how to calculate and avoid this penalty.

IRMAA

In this final section, we discuss the Income-Related Monthly Adjustment Amount (IRMAA) and its impact on Medicare Part D premiums. We explain how higher-income beneficiaries may be subject to additional premium surcharges based on their modified adjusted gross income (MAGI). We offer strategies for managing IRMAA and minimizing premium costs.

Overview of Part D

Medicare Part D is the prescription drug coverage component of Medicare, designed to help beneficiaries afford the medications they need to manage their health conditions. Part D plans are offered by private insurance companies approved by Medicare. These plans provide coverage for both brand-name and generic prescription drugs, helping to lower out-of-pocket costs for beneficiaries.

Part D plans work alongside Original Medicare (Parts A and B) and Medicare Advantage plans, providing an additional layer of coverage for prescription medications. Beneficiaries can choose from a variety of Part D plans, each offering different formularies (lists of covered drugs) and cost-sharing structures.

One key feature of Medicare Part D is the coverage gap, often referred to as the "donut hole." This is a temporary limit on what the drug plan will cover for prescription drug costs. Once a beneficiary reaches the initial coverage limit, they enter the coverage gap and are responsible for a larger share of their prescription drug costs until they reach the catastrophic coverage threshold.

Medicare Part D also provides access to catastrophic coverage, which offers additional financial protection for beneficiaries with high prescription drug costs. Once a beneficiary reaches the catastrophic coverage threshold, they pay only a small coinsurance or copayment for covered medications for the remainder of the year.

Overall, Medicare Part D plays a crucial role in helping beneficiaries afford necessary prescription medications and manage their health conditions effectively. By understanding how Part D works and enrolling in a plan that meets their needs, beneficiaries can access the medications they need while minimizing out-of-pocket costs.

Importance of Having Part D Coverage

Having Medicare Part D coverage is crucial for several reasons, each of which underscores the importance of enrolling in a Part D plan:

Access to Prescription Medications:

- Medicare Part D provides beneficiaries with access to a wide range of prescription medications, including both brand-name and generic drugs. Without Part D coverage, beneficiaries may face significant out-of-pocket costs for medications, potentially leading to delays or disruptions in treatment.

Financial Protection:

- Part D coverage helps beneficiaries afford prescription medications by covering a portion of the cost of their prescriptions. This financial assistance can be especially valuable for individuals on fixed incomes or with limited resources, helping to reduce the burden of prescription drug costs and prevent financial hardship.

Preventive Care and Disease Management:

- Prescription medications play a vital role in preventing and managing chronic health conditions, such as diabetes, heart disease, and hypertension. By ensuring access to necessary medications, Part D coverage supports beneficiaries in maintaining their health and well-being, reducing the risk of complications and hospitalizations.

Avoiding Late Enrollment Penalties:

- Enrolling in a Medicare Part D plan during your Initial Enrollment Period (IEP) or other applicable enrollment periods helps you avoid late enrollment penalties. If you go without creditable prescription drug coverage for a continuous period of 63 days or more after your IEP ends, you may incur a late enrollment penalty, resulting in higher premiums when you do enroll in a Part D plan.

Peace of Mind:

- Having Medicare Part D coverage provides beneficiaries with peace of mind, knowing that they have financial protection and access to necessary medications to manage their health conditions. With Part D coverage in place, beneficiaries can focus on their health and well-being without worrying about the cost of prescription medications.

Overall, Medicare Part D coverage is essential for ensuring access to prescription medications, financial protection, preventive care, and peace of mind for beneficiaries. By enrolling in a Part D plan that meets their needs, beneficiaries can effectively manage their health conditions and maintain their quality of life.

How to Enroll

Enrolling in a Medicare Part D prescription drug plan is a straightforward process, and there are several options available to beneficiaries:

Initial Enrollment Period (IEP):

- The Initial Enrollment Period (IEP) for Medicare Part D begins three months before your 65th birthday month and extends for three months after. During this seven-month period, you have the opportunity to enroll in a Part D plan for the first time without incurring late enrollment penalties.

Annual Enrollment Period (AEP):

- The Annual Enrollment Period (AEP), also known as the Medicare Open Enrollment Period, occurs each year from October 15th to

December 7th. During this time, you can enroll in a Part D plan for the first time, switch to a different Part D plan, or drop your current Part D coverage.

Special Enrollment Periods (SEPs):

- Special Enrollment Periods (SEPs) may be available to beneficiaries who experience certain qualifying events, such as moving to a new area with different plan options, losing other prescription drug coverage, or becoming eligible for Extra Help (low-income subsidy). SEPs allow you to enroll in or make changes to your Part D coverage outside of the Annual Enrollment Period.

To enroll in a Medicare Part D prescription drug plan, you can follow these steps:

Research Part D Plans:

- Begin by researching the Part D plans available in your area. You can use the Medicare Plan Finder tool on the Medicare website to compare plan options, including premiums, deductibles, copayments, and covered medications.

Consider Your Medication Needs:

- Evaluate your current prescription medication needs and preferences. Consider factors such as the medications you take regularly, their dosages, and whether they are covered by the Part D plans you are considering.

Compare Plan Costs and Coverage:

- Compare the costs and coverage benefits of different Part D plans to determine which plan best meets your medication needs and budget. Pay attention to factors such as monthly premiums, annual deductibles, copayments or coinsurance, and coverage for your specific medications.

Enroll Online, by Phone, or by Mail:

- Once you've chosen a Part D plan, you can enroll online through the Medicare website, by calling Medicare's toll-free number at 1-800-MEDICARE (1-800-633-4227), or by completing a paper enrollment form and mailing it to the plan provider.

Provide Necessary Information:

- When enrolling in a Part D plan, you'll need to provide certain personal information, such as your Medicare card number, date of birth, and contact information. You may also need to provide information about your current prescription drug coverage, if applicable.

Confirm Enrollment:

- After submitting your enrollment application, you should receive confirmation of your enrollment from the Part D plan provider. Review the details of your coverage, including your effective date of coverage, premium payment instructions, and any additional information provided by the plan.

By following these steps, beneficiaries can enroll in a Medicare Part D prescription drug plan that meets their medication needs and budget, ensuring access to necessary medications and financial protection against prescription drug costs. If you have questions or need assistance with enrollment, consider reaching out to a licensed insurance agent or Medicare counselor for personalized guidance.

Late Enrollment Penalty

The late enrollment penalty is a financial consequence that Medicare beneficiaries may incur if they do not enroll in a Medicare Part D prescription drug plan when first eligible and go without creditable prescription drug coverage for a continuous period of 63 days or more. Here's a detailed overview of the late enrollment penalty and how to avoid it:

Calculation of the Penalty:

- The late enrollment penalty is calculated by multiplying 1% of the "national base beneficiary premium" by the number of full months you were eligible for Part D coverage but did not enroll or have creditable coverage. The national base beneficiary premium may change each year and is used as a benchmark for calculating the penalty.

Addition to Monthly Premium:

- If you incur a late enrollment penalty, it will be added to your Medicare Part D premium and will continue to apply for as long as you have Medicare Part D coverage. The penalty amount may vary depending on how long you went without creditable prescription drug coverage and can result in higher monthly premiums.

Avoiding the Penalty:

- The best way to avoid the late enrollment penalty is to enroll in a Medicare Part D prescription drug plan during your Initial Enrollment Period (IEP) or other applicable enrollment periods. Your IEP begins three months before your 65th birthday month and extends for three months after. During this time, you have the opportunity to enroll in a Part D plan without incurring penalties.

Special Enrollment Periods:

- If you miss your Initial Enrollment Period or other applicable enrollment periods, you may still be able to enroll in a Part D plan without incurring a penalty if you qualify for a Special Enrollment Period (SEP). SEPs are available to beneficiaries who experience certain qualifying events, such as losing other prescription drug coverage or moving to a new area with different plan options.

Reviewing Creditable Coverage:

- If you have other prescription drug coverage, such as through an employer or union, it's essential to review whether your coverage is considered creditable. Creditable coverage means that your current prescription drug coverage is expected to pay, on average, at least as much as Medicare's standard prescription drug coverage. If your current coverage is creditable, you may be able to delay enrolling in a Part D plan without incurring a penalty.

By understanding the late enrollment penalty and taking proactive steps to enroll in Medicare Part D coverage during your Initial Enrollment Period or other applicable enrollment periods, you can avoid penalties and ensure access to affordable prescription medications. If you have questions or need assistance with enrollment, consider reaching out to a licensed insurance agent or Medicare counselor for personalized guidance.

IRMAA (Income-Related Monthly Adjustment Amount)

The Income-Related Monthly Adjustment Amount (IRMAA) is an additional premium that some Medicare beneficiaries may be required to pay for Part D prescription drug coverage, as well as for Medicare Part B (medical insurance) and Part C (Medicare Advantage) premiums. Here's a detailed overview of IRMAA and who it applies to:

Determining IRMAA:

- IRMAA is based on your modified adjusted gross income (MAGI) from two years ago, as reported to the Internal Revenue Service (IRS). The Social Security Administration (SSA) uses your MAGI to determine whether you'll pay an IRMAA and, if so, how much.

Income Thresholds:

- Medicare uses specific income thresholds to determine if you'll be subject to IRMAA. These thresholds vary depending on your filing status (individual or married filing jointly) and are adjusted annually for inflation. If your MAGI exceeds these thresholds, you may be subject to IRMAA.

IRMAA Tiers:

- IRMAA is calculated based on five income tiers. The higher your income, the higher your IRMAA. For Medicare Part D, the income thresholds and corresponding IRMAA amounts are as follows for individuals and married couples filing jointly (2023 figures):

- Tier 1 (Less than $91,000 for individuals, less than $182,000 for married couples): No IRMAA
- Tier 2 ($91,000 to $114,000 for individuals, $182,000 to $228,000 for married couples): IRMAA of $12.40 to $77.90 per month
- Tier 3 ($114,000 to $142,000 for individuals, $228,000 to $284,000 for married couples): IRMAA of $31.70 to $179.20 per month
- Tier 4 ($142,000 to $170,000 for individuals, $284,000 to $340,000 for married couples): IRMAA of $51.20 to $280.90 per month
- Tier 5 (Above $170,000 for individuals, above $340,000 for married couples): IRMAA of $70.70 to $384.20 per month

Who IRMAA Applies To:

- IRMAA applies to Medicare beneficiaries with higher incomes, including individuals with a MAGI of $91,000 or more and married couples filing jointly with a MAGI of $182,000 or more. It's important to note that IRMAA applies to both Medicare Part D and Part B premiums, as well as to Medicare Advantage premiums for beneficiaries who choose those plans.

Payment of IRMAA:

- If you're subject to IRMAA, you'll receive a notice from the SSA informing you of the additional amount you'll need to pay for your Medicare premiums. This amount is typically deducted from your Social Security benefits or billed directly to you if you're not receiving Social Security benefits.

Understanding IRMAA and its income thresholds can help Medicare beneficiaries anticipate and plan for potential additional premium costs. If you have questions about IRMAA or need assistance with understanding your Medicare premiums, consider reaching out to the Social Security Administration or a licensed insurance agent for personalized guidance.

Frequently Asked Questions

Medicare beneficiaries often have questions about Medicare Part D prescription drug coverage as they navigate their healthcare options. Here are some common questions and answers to help clarify Part D coverage:

What is Medicare Part D, and how does it work?

- Medicare Part D is the prescription drug coverage component of Medicare, offered through private insurance companies approved by Medicare. Part D plans help beneficiaries afford prescription medications by providing coverage for both brand-name and generic drugs. Beneficiaries pay a monthly premium, annual deductible, and copayments or coinsurance for their medications.

How do I enroll in a Medicare Part D plan?

- You can enroll in a Medicare Part D plan during your Initial Enrollment Period (IEP), which begins three months before your 65th birthday month and extends for three months after. You can also enroll during the Annual Enrollment Period (AEP) from October 15th to December 7th each year. To enroll, you can use the Medicare Plan Finder tool on the Medicare website, call Medicare's toll-free number, or contact a licensed insurance agent.

What medications are covered by Medicare Part D?

- Medicare Part D plans cover a wide range of prescription medications, including both brand-name and generic drugs. Each Part D plan has a formulary, or list of covered drugs, which may vary depending on the plan. It's essential to review a plan's formulary to ensure that your medications are covered before enrolling.

Are there any penalties for not enrolling in Medicare Part D?

- Yes, if you don't enroll in a Medicare Part D plan when you're first eligible and go without creditable prescription drug coverage for a continuous period of 63 days or more, you may incur a late enrollment penalty. This penalty is added to your monthly premium and can result in higher costs for as long as you have Part D coverage.

What is the Medicare Part D "donut hole," and how does it affect coverage?

- The Medicare Part D "donut hole" is a temporary limit on what your Part D plan will cover for prescription drug costs. Once you reach the initial coverage limit, you enter the coverage gap, where you're responsible for a larger share of your prescription drug costs. However, the coverage gap is gradually closing due to changes in healthcare legislation.

How can I lower my out-of-pocket costs for prescription medications with Medicare Part D?

- There are several strategies to lower out-of-pocket costs for prescription medications with Medicare Part D, such as choosing generic drugs when available, using preferred pharmacies, and utilizing medication therapy management services offered by your

Part D plan. You can also explore programs like Extra Help for assistance with prescription drug costs if you have limited income and resources.

These are just a few of the common questions Medicare beneficiaries have about Medicare Part D prescription drug coverage. If you have additional questions or need personalized assistance, consider reaching out to a licensed insurance agent or Medicare counselor for guidance.

5

Other Important Information To Know

This chapter serves as a comprehensive guide for Medicare members, providing essential information that may not have been covered in previous chapters. It offers insights into valuable resources, navigating Medicaid and Extra Help programs, understanding Long-Term Care (LTC), managing employer coverage past 65, familiarizing with common election periods, interpreting the Annual Notice of Change letter, and safeguarding against scams.

Helpful Resources

This section offers a compilation of valuable resources available to Medicare members. It includes information on reputable websites, helplines, and government agencies that provide assistance with Medicare-related questions and concerns. Additionally, it highlights community organizations and support groups that offer guidance and advocacy for Medicare beneficiaries.

Medicaid and Extra Help

Here, we provide an overview of Medicaid and the Extra Help

program, which offer financial assistance to eligible individuals with limited income and resources. We explain the eligibility criteria for these programs and how beneficiaries can apply for assistance with Medicare premiums, deductibles, and prescription drug costs.

Long-Term Care (LTC)

In this section, we discuss the importance of planning for long-term care needs and the various options available for financing long-term care services. We provide an overview of long-term care insurance, Medicaid coverage for nursing home care, and alternative care options such as home health care and assisted living facilities.

Keeping Employer Coverage Past 65

This section addresses the options available to Medicare beneficiaries who wish to maintain employer-sponsored health coverage after turning 65. We discuss the coordination of benefits between Medicare and employer coverage, including considerations for enrolling in Medicare Part A and delaying enrollment in Part B.

Common Election Periods

Here, we outline the various election periods that Medicare beneficiaries may encounter, such as the Initial Enrollment Period (IEP), Annual Enrollment Period (AEP), Special Enrollment Periods (SEPs), and Medicare Advantage Open Enrollment Period (MA OEP). We explain the purpose of each period and the opportunities for beneficiaries to make changes to their Medicare coverage.

Annual Notice of Change Letter

This section educates beneficiaries about the Annual Notice of Change (ANOC) letter, which Medicare Advantage and Medicare Part D plans send each year to notify members of changes to their plan's benefits, premiums, and provider networks. We provide guidance on how to review and interpret the ANOC letter to make informed decisions about plan coverage.

How to Identify Scams and Avoid Them

In the final section, we offer tips and strategies for recognizing and avoiding Medicare-related scams. We discuss common scams targeting Medicare beneficiaries, such as fraudulent phone calls, emails, and advertisements, and provide guidance on how to protect personal information and report suspected scams to the appropriate authorities.

Helpful Resources

Navigating Medicare can sometimes be complex, but there are numerous resources available to assist beneficiaries in understanding their coverage and maximizing their benefits. Here are some helpful resources that Medicare members can access:

Medicare.gov:

- The official Medicare website, Medicare.gov, is a valuable resource for beneficiaries seeking information about their coverage options, enrollment periods, and benefits. The website offers interactive tools, such as the Medicare Plan Finder and Coverage Wizard, to help beneficiaries compare plans and find the coverage that best meets their needs.

Medicare Helpline:

- Medicare offers a toll-free helpline at 1-800-MEDICARE (1-800-633-4227), where beneficiaries can speak to a representative for assistance with their Medicare-related questions and concerns. The helpline is available 24 hours a day, seven days a week, and provides support in multiple languages.

State Health Insurance Assistance Program (SHIP):

- The State Health Insurance Assistance Program (SHIP) provides free, unbiased counseling and assistance to Medicare beneficiaries and their families. SHIP counselors can help beneficiaries understand their Medicare benefits, compare coverage options, and navigate Medicare enrollment and appeals processes.

Social Security Administration (SSA):

- The Social Security Administration (SSA) oversees Medicare enrollment and administration, including processing applications for Medicare benefits and issuing Medicare cards. Beneficiaries can visit the SSA website or local SSA offices for assistance with Medicare-related inquiries and concerns.

Local Area Agencies on Aging (AAA):

- Local Area Agencies on Aging (AAA) offer a range of services and programs to support older adults and Medicare beneficiaries in their communities. AAA offices can provide information and assistance with Medicare enrollment, health insurance counseling, and access to community resources and services.

Medicare & You Handbook:

- The "Medicare & You" handbook is an official guide published annually by Medicare, providing detailed information about Medicare benefits, coverage options, enrollment periods, and preventive services. Beneficiaries receive a copy of the handbook each year and can also access it online via the Medicare website.

Medicare Advantage and Part D Plans:

- Medicare beneficiaries can contact their Medicare Advantage or Part D plan providers directly for assistance with plan-specific inquiries, such as coverage details, formularies, and network providers. Plan representatives can provide personalized guidance and support to help beneficiaries understand and utilize their plan benefits effectively.

By utilizing these resources, Medicare beneficiaries can gain a better understanding of their coverage options, access support and guidance when needed, and make informed decisions to maximize their Medicare benefits.

Medicaid and Extra Help

Medicaid and the Extra Help program (also known as the Low-Income Subsidy) are two important assistance programs that provide financial support to eligible individuals with limited income and resources, helping them afford healthcare costs, including Medicare expenses. Here's a detailed description of each program and how they coordinate with Medicare:

Medicaid:

- Medicaid is a joint federal and state program that provides comprehensive healthcare coverage to eligible individuals and families with low income and limited resources. Medicaid benefits vary by state but typically include services such as doctor visits, hospital care, prescription drugs, and long-term care. In some states, Medicaid also offers coverage for Medicare premiums, deductibles, coinsurance, and copayments, effectively reducing out-of-pocket costs for Medicare beneficiaries with limited financial means.

Extra Help (Low-Income Subsidy):

- The Extra Help program, also known as the Low-Income Subsidy (LIS), is a federal program administered by the Social Security Administration (SSA) that helps Medicare beneficiaries with limited income and resources afford prescription drug costs under Medicare Part D. Extra Help helps with premiums, deductibles, and copayments for Medicare Part D prescription drug plans, making medications more affordable for eligible beneficiaries. The level of Extra Help a beneficiary receives depends on their income and resources, with higher levels of assistance available to those with lower income and assets.

Both Medicaid and Extra Help coordinate with Medicare to provide financial assistance to eligible beneficiaries and help cover healthcare costs. Medicaid may help with Medicare premiums, deductibles, coinsurance, and copayments, as well as additional benefits such as dental, vision, and long-term care services. Extra Help specifically targets prescription drug costs, reducing out-of-pocket expenses for Medicare Part D beneficiaries. Beneficiaries who qualify for both Medicaid and Extra Help may receive comprehensive coverage for their healthcare needs, including prescription medications, at little to no cost.

Eligibility for Medicaid and Extra Help is based on income and resources, and beneficiaries must meet specific criteria to qualify for assistance. Individuals can apply for both programs separately through their state Medicaid agency and the Social Security Administration, respectively. By coordinating with Medicare, Medicaid and Extra Help play a crucial role in ensuring access to affordable healthcare for vulnerable populations, including older adults and individuals with disabilities.

Long-Term Care (LTC)

Long-term care (LTC) services, including assistance with activities of daily living such as bathing, dressing, and meal preparation, are not typically covered by Medicare. However, there are several options available for Medicare beneficiaries to obtain coverage for long-term care services. Here's an explanation of how beneficiaries can access LTC coverage:

Long-Term Care Insurance:

- Long-term care insurance is a private insurance policy specifically designed to cover the costs of long-term care services, including skilled nursing care, assisted living facilities, and home health care. Beneficiaries can purchase long-term care insurance policies from private insurance companies, with coverage options and premiums varying based on factors such as age, health status, and desired benefits. It's essential for beneficiaries to research different insurance options and carefully review policy terms and coverage limits to ensure they select a policy that meets their long-term care needs.

Medicaid Coverage for Long-Term Care:

- Medicaid is the largest payer of long-term care services in the United States and provides coverage for eligible individuals who require assistance with activities of daily living and meet certain income and asset criteria. Medicaid covers a wide range of long-term care services, including nursing home care, home health care, and personal care services. To qualify for Medicaid coverage for long-term care, beneficiaries must meet specific eligibility requirements set by their state, which typically include income and asset limits. Individuals can apply for Medicaid coverage through their state Medicaid agency, and eligibility determinations are based on financial need and functional eligibility criteria.

Veterans Administration (VA) Benefits:

- Military veterans may be eligible for long-term care benefits through the Veterans Administration (VA), including coverage for nursing home care, assisted living facilities, and home-based care services. The VA offers a variety of long-term care programs and services for eligible veterans, dependents, and survivors, with eligibility criteria varying based on factors such as military service history, disability status, and income. Veterans can contact their local VA medical center or regional VA office for information about available long-term care benefits and how to apply for assistance.

Personal Savings and Assets:

- Some beneficiaries may choose to self-fund their long-term care expenses using personal savings, retirement accounts, and other assets. Setting aside funds in advance or purchasing annuities or other financial products specifically designed for long-term care planning can help individuals prepare for future care needs and mitigate the financial burden of long-term care services. It's essential for beneficiaries to work with a financial advisor or elder law attorney to develop a comprehensive long-term care plan that aligns with their financial goals and priorities.

By exploring these options for obtaining coverage for long-term care services, Medicare beneficiaries can proactively plan for their future care needs and ensure access to quality long-term care services when necessary. It's recommended for individuals to research and evaluate different coverage options, seek guidance from trusted advisors, and make informed decisions based on their individual circumstances and preferences.

Keeping Employer Coverage Past 65

Many Medicare beneficiaries may have access to employer-sponsored health coverage through their own or their spouse's employment past the age of 65. In this section, we explore the options available to beneficiaries who wish to maintain their employer coverage and provide guidance on coordinating benefits with Medicare:

Coordination of Benefits:

- When individuals are eligible for both Medicare and employer-sponsored health coverage, coordination of benefits ensures that healthcare expenses are covered appropriately. Medicare generally becomes the primary payer if the employer coverage is from a small employer (20 employees or less) or if the individual is retired. However, if the employer coverage is from a large employer (more than 20 employees) and the individual is actively working, the employer coverage remains the primary payer, and Medicare acts as secondary insurance.

Enrolling in Medicare Part A:

- Most individuals are eligible for premium-free Medicare Part A (hospital insurance) at age 65, even if they continue working and have employer coverage. It's generally advisable for beneficiaries to enroll in Medicare Part A when first eligible, as it may provide additional coverage and help cover costs not covered by employer-sponsored insurance, such as hospital stays and skilled nursing facility care.

Delaying Enrollment in Medicare Part B:

- For beneficiaries who have credible employer-sponsored health coverage, particularly from a large employer, they may choose to delay enrolling in Medicare Part B (medical insurance) without facing penalties. As long as the individual or their spouse is actively working and covered under a group health plan based on current employment, they can delay Part B enrollment without penalty until the employment or coverage ends, whichever comes first. It's essential for beneficiaries to verify with their employer whether their coverage is considered credible before making decisions about delaying Part B enrollment.

Special Enrollment Period (SEP):

- If beneficiaries decide to delay Medicare Part B enrollment due to having credible employer coverage, they have a Special Enrollment Period (SEP) to enroll in Part B without penalty once the employer coverage ends. The SEP lasts for eight months, beginning the month after employment or coverage ends, whichever comes first. Beneficiaries should be mindful of the SEP timeframe and enroll in Part B promptly to avoid coverage gaps and potential penalties.

Understanding Coverage Options:

- Beneficiaries should carefully review their employer-sponsored health coverage, including costs, benefits, and provider networks, to understand how it complements Medicare. They should also consider factors such as retiree health benefits, COBRA coverage, and retiree health savings accounts (HSAs) when making decisions about Medicare enrollment and employer coverage.

By understanding the options available for maintaining employer-sponsored health coverage past the age of 65 and coordinating benefits with Medicare, beneficiaries can make informed decisions about their healthcare coverage and ensure seamless access to healthcare services. It's recommended for individuals to consult with their employer's benefits administrator, Medicare counselor, or insurance agent for personalized guidance based on their individual circumstances and needs.

Common Election Periods

Medicare beneficiaries may encounter various election periods throughout the year that allow them to make changes to their Medicare coverage based on their needs and circumstances. In this section, we outline the purpose of each election period and the opportunities they provide for beneficiaries to modify their Medicare coverage:

Initial Enrollment Period (IEP):

- The Initial Enrollment Period (IEP) is the seven-month period that begins three months before the month an individual turns 65, includes the month of their 65th birthday, and extends for three months after. During the IEP, beneficiaries can enroll in Medicare Parts A and B, as well as Medicare Advantage and standalone Medicare Part D prescription drug plans.

Annual Enrollment Period (AEP):

• The Annual Enrollment Period (AEP), also known as the Fall Open Enrollment Period, occurs annually from October 15th to December 7th. During this period, beneficiaries can make changes to their Medicare coverage, including switching Medicare Advantage plans, joining or leaving Medicare Part D prescription drug plans, and returning to Original Medicare from a Medicare Advantage plan.

Special Enrollment Periods (SEPs):

• Special Enrollment Periods (SEPs) are available to beneficiaries who experience qualifying life events that affect their Medicare coverage. Examples of qualifying events include moving to a new address, losing employer-sponsored health coverage, becoming eligible for Medicaid, or being affected by a natural disaster or public health emergency. SEPs allow beneficiaries to make changes to their Medicare coverage outside of the standard enrollment periods.

Medicare Advantage Open Enrollment Period (MA OEP):

• The Medicare Advantage Open Enrollment Period (MA OEP) occurs annually from January 1st to March 31st. During this period, beneficiaries enrolled in Medicare Advantage plans have the opportunity to make a one-time change to a different Medicare Advantage plan or switch to Original Medicare with or without a standalone Part D prescription drug plan. Beneficiaries cannot use this period to enroll in Part D if they are in Original Medicare.

Understanding these common election periods is essential for beneficiaries to take advantage of opportunities to make changes to their Medicare coverage as needed. By staying informed about enrollment periods and eligibility criteria for special enrollment opportunities, beneficiaries can ensure they have the coverage that best meets their healthcare needs throughout the year. It's recommended for individuals to review their Medicare coverage annually and explore available options to make informed decisions about their healthcare coverage.

Annual Notice of Change Letter

The Annual Notice of Change (ANOC) letter is an important communication that Medicare Advantage and Medicare Part D plans send to their members each year. In this section, we educate beneficiaries about the purpose of the ANOC letter and provide guidance on how to review and interpret its contents to make informed decisions about their plan coverage:

Purpose of the ANOC Letter:

- The ANOC letter serves as a notification from Medicare Advantage and Medicare Part D plans to their members about any changes to the plan's benefits, premiums, provider networks, or coverage rules for the upcoming plan year. It is sent annually before the Annual Enrollment Period (AEP) to ensure beneficiaries have time to review the changes and make informed decisions about their coverage options.

The ANOC letter typically includes important information such as:

- Changes to plan benefits: Any changes to covered services, copayments, coinsurance, or deductibles.
- Premium changes: Any changes to the monthly premium for the plan.
- Provider network changes: Any changes to the network of doctors, hospitals, pharmacies, or other healthcare providers that participate in the plan.
- Prescription drug formulary changes: Any changes to the list of covered medications (formulary), including additions, removals, or changes to coverage tiers.

When reviewing the ANOC letter, beneficiaries should pay close attention to any changes that may affect their healthcare coverage and costs for the upcoming year. It's essential to:

- Compare plan benefits: Review changes to covered services, copayments, and deductibles to assess how they may impact your healthcare needs and expenses.
- Check premium changes: Determine if there are any changes to the plan's monthly premium and evaluate whether the cost is still affordable.
- Confirm provider network changes: Ensure that your preferred doctors, hospitals, pharmacies, and other healthcare providers remain in-network to avoid unexpected out-of-pocket costs.
- Review prescription drug coverage: Check for any changes to the plan's prescription drug formulary to ensure that your medications will continue to be covered at an affordable cost.

By carefully reviewing and interpreting the ANOC letter, beneficiaries can make informed decisions about their Medicare Advantage or Medicare Part D coverage for the upcoming plan year. It's recommended for individuals to take the time to thoroughly review the letter, compare their options, and consider any changes to their healthcare needs when selecting a plan during the Annual Enrollment Period (AEP). Additionally, beneficiaries can contact their plan's customer service department or seek assistance from a Medicare counselor if they have questions or need further clarification about the ANOC letter or their plan options.

How to Identify Scams and Avoid Them

Protecting oneself from Medicare-related scams is crucial for beneficiaries to safeguard their personal information and financial well-being. In this section, we provide tips and strategies for recognizing and avoiding scams targeting Medicare beneficiaries, along with guidance on how to protect personal information and report suspected scams to the appropriate authorities:

Be Vigilant:

- Stay alert and be cautious of unsolicited phone calls, emails, letters, or advertisements claiming to be from Medicare or government agencies. Scammers often use fear tactics or promises of free services or benefits to deceive unsuspecting beneficiaries.

Know the Red Flags:

- Common red flags of Medicare scams include requests for personal information such as Medicare or Social Security numbers, demands for payment or enrollment fees, pressure to make immediate decisions, and offers that seem too good to be true.

Verify Identity:

- Before providing any personal or financial information, verify the identity of the individual or organization contacting you. Legitimate Medicare representatives will never ask for personal information over the phone or email without prior authorization.

Guard Personal Information:

- Never share your Medicare, Social Security, or bank account numbers with unknown individuals or entities. Be cautious when providing personal information, and only disclose it to trusted sources or authorized healthcare providers.

Review Medicare Statements:

- Regularly review your Medicare Summary Notice (MSN) or Explanation of Benefits (EOB) statements for any discrepancies or suspicious charges. Report any unauthorized or unfamiliar charges to Medicare immediately.

Protect Against Identity Theft:

- Safeguard your personal information by shredding documents containing sensitive data, securing your Medicare card, and using strong, unique passwords for online accounts. Be cautious when sharing personal information online or on social media platforms.

Report Suspected Scams:

- If you suspect you've been targeted by a Medicare scam or fraudulent activity, report it immediately to the appropriate authorities. Contact Medicare's fraud hotline at 1-800-MEDICARE (1-800-633-4227) or report online through the Medicare website. You can also report scams to the Federal Trade Commission (FTC) at ftc.gov/complaint or call 1-877-FTC-HELP (1-877-382-4357).

By following these tips and strategies, Medicare beneficiaries can protect themselves against scams and fraudulent activities, minimize the risk of identity theft and financial fraud, and ensure a safe and secure healthcare experience. It's essential to stay informed, remain vigilant, and report any suspicious activity promptly to help combat Medicare fraud and protect the integrity of the Medicare program.

6

Conclusion

As we conclude this essential guide to mastering Medicare, it's crucial to reflect on the wealth of information and insights we've explored together. Throughout the chapters, we've embarked on a journey to demystify the complexities of Medicare, empowering you with the knowledge and tools needed to navigate the healthcare system with confidence and clarity.

From understanding the fundamental components of Original Medicare to exploring the intricacies of Medicare Advantage, Medigap, and Part D prescription drug coverage, each chapter has provided invaluable guidance tailored to your unique needs as a Medicare beneficiary. We've delved into the nuances of enrollment periods, coverage options, and supplemental programs, equipping you with the expertise to make informed decisions about your healthcare coverage.

In the first chapter, we laid the groundwork by providing a comprehensive overview of Medicare and its various parts, ensuring a solid understanding of the foundational elements that form the backbone of your healthcare coverage. We then delved into the specifics of each component, breaking down complex concepts into digestible insights that empower you to maximize your coverage while minimizing confusion.

Throughout the chapters, we've emphasized the importance of proactive planning and informed decision-making, urging you to take an active role in managing your healthcare journey. Whether it's exploring options for long-term care, understanding the nuances of coordination between Medicare and employer-sponsored coverage, or safeguarding against Medicare-related scams, we've equipped you with the knowledge and resources to navigate each aspect of your healthcare experience with confidence and resilience.

As we've journeyed through the intricacies of Medicare, it's important to recognize the significance of this milestone in your healthcare journey. Turning 65 or enrolling in Medicare due to a qualifying disability marks a pivotal moment in your life, and mastering Medicare is not just about understanding coverage—it's about taking control of your health and well-being, ensuring you have access to the care and support you need to thrive.

We've also highlighted the importance of staying informed and remaining vigilant in the face of evolving healthcare landscapes and emerging challenges. From keeping abreast of changes to your plan's benefits and premiums through the Annual Notice of Change (ANOC) letter to protecting yourself against Medicare scams and fraudulent activities, we've underscored the importance of knowledge and awareness in safeguarding your healthcare journey.

As you embark on your Medicare journey, remember that you are not alone. From the invaluable support of family and friends to the expertise of healthcare professionals and trusted advisors, there is a wealth of resources and support available to guide you every step of the way. Don't hesitate to reach out for assistance or seek clarification whenever needed—your health and well-being are paramount, and there are dedicated individuals and organizations committed to helping you navigate the complexities of Medicare with ease and confidence.

In closing, I want to extend my heartfelt gratitude to you, the reader, for entrusting me as your guide on this journey to mastering Medicare. It has been an honor and a privilege to accompany you on this transformative exploration of healthcare, and I hope that the knowledge and insights gained will serve you well as you navigate the intricacies of Medicare and embark on a path to lifelong health and wellness.

Remember, mastering Medicare is not just about understanding coverage—it's about empowering yourself to take control of your health, advocate for your needs, and embrace the opportunities that lie ahead. May your Medicare journey be filled with empowerment, resilience, and the unwavering determination to live your best life, today and always.

With warmest regards and best wishes for your health and happiness,

M.T Edward.